MAKE IT STOP

Headache Tracker

MAKE IT STOP

MONTHLY TOTAL

MONTH

MONDAY	TUESDAY	WEDNESDAY	THURSDAY	FRIDAY	SATURDAY	SUNDAY

DATE________________________

DURATION________________________

WHERE IT HURTS

INTENSITY

PAIN CHARACTERISTICS

TREATMENT

FACTORS

SLEEP

CAFFEINE

ALCOHOL

WATER

FOOD

WEATHER

OTHER FACTORS

NOTES

DATE

DURATION

INTENSITY

PAIN CHARACTERISTICS

TREATMENT

WHERE IT HURTS

FACTORS

SLEEP

CAFFEINE

ALCOHOL

WATER

FOOD

WEATHER

NOTES

OTHER FACTORS

DATE_____________________________________

DURATION_____________________________

WHERE IT HURTS

INTENSITY

PAIN CHARACTERISTICS

TREATMENT

FACTORS

SLEEP

CAFFEINE

ALCOHOL

WATER

FOOD

WEATHER

OTHER FACTORS

NOTES

DATE_____________________

DURATION_____________________

WHERE IT HURTS

INTENSITY

PAIN CHARACTERISTICS

TREATMENT

FACTORS

SLEEP

CAFFEINE

ALCOHOL

WATER

FOOD

WEATHER

OTHER FACTORS

NOTES

FACTORS

SLEEP

CAFFEINE

ALCOHOL

WATER

FOOD

WEATHER

OTHER FACTORS

NOTES

DATE________________________
DURATION________________________
INTENSITY
PAIN CHARACTERISTICS
TREATMENT
WHERE IT HURTS
FACTORS
SLEEP
CAFFEINE
ALCOHOL
WATER
FOOD
WEATHER
OTHER FACTORS
NOTES

DATE
DURATION
INTENSITY
PAIN CHARACTERISTICS
TREATMENT
WHERE IT HURTS
FACTORS
SLEEP
CAFFEINE
ALCOHOL
WATER
FOOD
WEATHER
OTHER FACTORS
NOTES

DATE
DURATION
INTENSITY
PAIN CHARACTERISTICS
TREATMENT
WHERE IT HURTS
FACTORS
SLEEP
OTHER FACTORS
CAFFEINE
ALCOHOL
WATER
FOOD
WEATHER
NOTES

DATE

DURATION

INTENSITY

PAIN CHARACTERISTICS

TREATMENT

WHERE IT HURTS

FACTORS

SLEEP

CAFFEINE

ALCOHOL

WATER

FOOD

WEATHER

OTHER FACTORS

NOTES

DATE_______________________

DURATION_______________________

INTENSITY

PAIN CHARACTERISTICS

TREATMENT

WHERE IT HURTS

FACTORS

SLEEP

CAFFEINE

ALCOHOL

WATER

FOOD

WEATHER

OTHER FACTORS

NOTES

DATE___________________

DURATION___________________

WHERE IT HURTS

INTENSITY

PAIN CHARACTERISTICS

TREATMENT

FACTORS

SLEEP

CAFFEINE

ALCOHOL

WATER

FOOD

WEATHER

OTHER FACTORS

NOTES

DATE
DURATION
INTENSITY
PAIN CHARACTERISTICS
TREATMENT
WHERE IT HURTS
FACTORS
SLEEP
OTHER FACTORS
CAFFEINE
ALCOHOL
WATER
FOOD
WEATHER
NOTES

DATE______________________

DURATION__________________________

WHERE IT HURTS

INTENSITY

PAIN CHARACTERISTICS

TREATMENT

FACTORS

SLEEP

CAFFEINE

ALCOHOL

WATER

FOOD

WEATHER

OTHER FACTORS

NOTES

DATE_______________________

DURATION_______________________

WHERE IT HURTS

INTENSITY

PAIN CHARACTERISTICS

TREATMENT

FACTORS

SLEEP

CAFFEINE

ALCOHOL

WATER

FOOD

WEATHER

OTHER FACTORS

NOTES

DATE_____________________ DURATION_____________________

WHERE IT HURTS

INTENSITY

PAIN CHARACTERISTICS

TREATMENT

FACTORS

SLEEP

CAFFEINE

ALCOHOL

WATER

FOOD

WEATHER

OTHER FACTORS

NOTES

DATE________________

DATE________________

DURATION________________

WHERE IT HURTS

INTENSITY

PAIN CHARACTERISTICS

TREATMENT

FACTORS

SLEEP

CAFFEINE

ALCOHOL

WATER

FOOD

WEATHER

OTHER FACTORS

NOTES

DATE
DURATION
INTENSITY
PAIN CHARACTERISTICS
TREATMENT
WHERE IT HURTS
FACTORS
SLEEP
CAFFEINE
ALCOHOL
WATER
FOOD
WEATHER
OTHER FACTORS
NOTES

DATE

DURATION

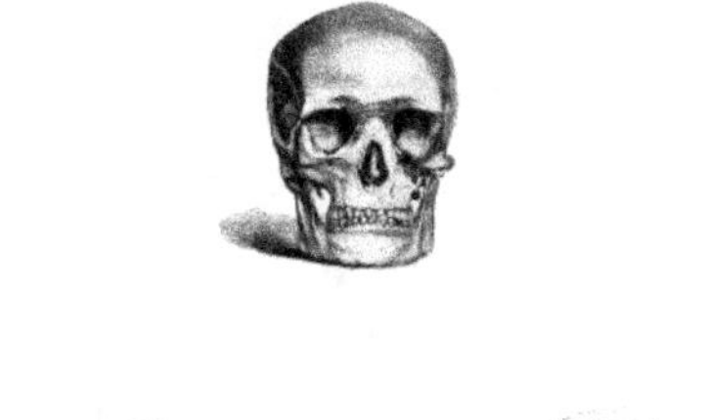

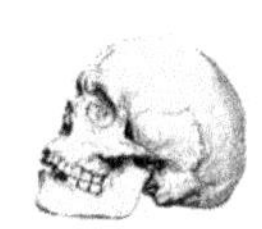

WHERE IT HURTS

INTENSITY

PAIN CHARACTERISTICS

TREATMENT

FACTORS

SLEEP

CAFFEINE

ALCOHOL

WATER

FOOD

WEATHER

OTHER FACTORS

NOTES

DATE

DURATION

INTENSITY

PAIN CHARACTERISTICS

TREATMENT

WHERE IT HURTS

FACTORS

SLEEP

CAFFEINE

ALCOHOL

WATER

FOOD

WEATHER

OTHER FACTORS

NOTES

DATE________________________

DURATION________________________

WHERE IT HURTS

INTENSITY

PAIN CHARACTERISTICS

TREATMENT

FACTORS

SLEEP

CAFFEINE

ALCOHOL

WATER

FOOD

WEATHER

OTHER FACTORS

NOTES

DATE_______________________

DURATION_______________________

INTENSITY

PAIN CHARACTERISTICS

TREATMENT

WHERE IT HURTS

FACTORS

SLEEP

CAFFEINE

ALCOHOL

WATER

FOOD

WEATHER

OTHER FACTORS

NOTES

DATE

DURATION

INTENSITY

PAIN CHARACTERISTICS

TREATMENT

FACTORS

SLEEP

CAFFEINE

ALCOHOL

WATER

FOOD

WEATHER

OTHER FACTORS

NOTES

DATE________________________

DURATION________________________

INTENSITY

PAIN CHARACTERISTICS

TREATMENT

FACTORS

SLEEP

CAFFEINE

ALCOHOL

WATER

FOOD

WEATHER

OTHER FACTORS

NOTES

DATE

DURATION

INTENSITY

PAIN CHARACTERISTICS

TREATMENT

FACTORS

SLEEP

CAFFEINE

ALCOHOL

WATER

FOOD

WEATHER

OTHER FACTORS

NOTES

DATE

DURATION

INTENSITY

PAIN CHARACTERISTICS

TREATMENT

WHERE IT HURTS

FACTORS

SLEEP

CAFFEINE

ALCOHOL

WATER

FOOD

WEATHER

OTHER FACTORS

NOTES

DATE______________________

DURATION______________________

INTENSITY

PAIN CHARACTERISTICS

TREATMENT

WHERE IT HURTS

FACTORS

SLEEP

CAFFEINE

ALCOHOL

WATER

FOOD

WEATHER

OTHER FACTORS

NOTES

DATE______________________
DURATION______________________

WHERE IT HURTS

INTENSITY

PAIN CHARACTERISTICS

TREATMENT

FACTORS

SLEEP
CAFFEINE
ALCOHOL
WATER
FOOD
WEATHER

OTHER FACTORS

NOTES

DATE

DURATION

INTENSITY

PAIN CHARACTERISTICS

TREATMENT

WHERE IT HURTS

FACTORS

SLEEP

CAFFEINE

ALCOHOL

WATER

FOOD

WEATHER

OTHER FACTORS

NOTES

DATE
DURATION
INTENSITY
PAIN CHARACTERISTICS
TREATMENT
WHERE IT HURTS
FACTORS
SLEEP
CAFFEINE
ALCOHOL
WATER
FOOD
WEATHER
OTHER FACTORS
NOTES

DATE

DURATION

WHERE IT HURTS

INTENSITY

PAIN CHARACTERISTICS

TREATMENT

FACTORS

SLEEP

CAFFEINE

ALCOHOL

WATER

FOOD

WEATHER

OTHER FACTORS

NOTES

DATE

DURATION

INTENSITY

PAIN CHARACTERISTICS

TREATMENT

WHERE IT HURTS

FACTORS

SLEEP

CAFFEINE

ALCOHOL

WATER

FOOD

WEATHER

OTHER FACTORS

NOTES

DATE

DURATION

WHERE IT HURTS

INTENSITY

PAIN CHARACTERISTICS

TREATMENT

FACTORS

SLEEP

CAFFEINE

ALCOHOL

WATER

FOOD

WEATHER

OTHER FACTORS

NOTES

DATE
DURATION
INTENSITY
PAIN CHARACTERISTICS
TREATMENT
WHERE IT HURTS
FACTORS
SLEEP
CAFFEINE
ALCOHOL
WATER
FOOD
WEATHER
OTHER FACTORS
NOTES

DATE

DURATION

INTENSITY

PAIN CHARACTERISTICS

TREATMENT

FACTORS

SLEEP

CAFFEINE

ALCOHOL

WATER

FOOD

WEATHER

OTHER FACTORS

NOTES

DATE _______________________

DURATION _______________________

WHERE IT HURTS

INTENSITY

PAIN CHARACTERISTICS

TREATMENT

FACTORS

SLEEP

CAFFEINE

ALCOHOL

WATER

FOOD

WEATHER

NOTES

OTHER FACTORS

DATE

DURATION

INTENSITY

PAIN CHARACTERISTICS

TREATMENT

WHERE IT HURTS

FACTORS

SLEEP

CAFFEINE

ALCOHOL

WATER

FOOD

WEATHER

OTHER FACTORS

NOTES

FACTORS

SLEEP	OTHER FACTORS
CAFFEINE	
ALCOHOL	
WATER	
FOOD	
WEATHER	

NOTES

DATE

DURATION

INTENSITY

PAIN CHARACTERISTICS

TREATMENT

WHERE IT HURTS

FACTORS

SLEEP

CAFFEINE

ALCOHOL

WATER

FOOD

WEATHER

OTHER FACTORS

NOTES

DATE
DURATION
INTENSITY
PAIN CHARACTERISTICS
TREATMENT
WHERE IT HURTS
FACTORS
SLEEP
CAFFEINE
ALCOHOL
WATER
FOOD
WEATHER
OTHER FACTORS
NOTES

FACTORS

SLEEP

CAFFEINE

ALCOHOL

WATER

FOOD

WEATHER

OTHER FACTORS

NOTES

DATE

DURATION

INTENSITY

PAIN CHARACTERISTICS

TREATMENT

WHERE IT HURTS

FACTORS

SLEEP

CAFFEINE

ALCOHOL

WATER

FOOD

WEATHER

OTHER FACTORS

NOTES

DATE
DURATION
INTENSITY
PAIN CHARACTERISTICS
TREATMENT
WHERE IT HURTS
FACTORS
SLEEP
CAFFEINE
ALCOHOL
WATER
FOOD
WEATHER
OTHER FACTORS
NOTES

DATE

DURATION

INTENSITY

PAIN CHARACTERISTICS

TREATMENT

WHERE IT HURTS

FACTORS

SLEEP

CAFFEINE

ALCOHOL

WATER

FOOD

WEATHER

OTHER FACTORS

NOTES

DATE

DURATION

INTENSITY

PAIN CHARACTERISTICS

TREATMENT

WHERE IT HURTS

FACTORS

SLEEP

CAFFEINE

ALCOHOL

WATER

FOOD

WEATHER

OTHER FACTORS

NOTES

DATE

DURATION

INTENSITY

PAIN CHARACTERISTICS

TREATMENT

WHERE IT HURTS

FACTORS

SLEEP

OTHER FACTORS

CAFFEINE

ALCOHOL

WATER

FOOD

WEATHER

NOTES

DATE______________________________

DURATION______________________

INTENSITY

PAIN CHARACTERISTICS

TREATMENT

WHERE IT HURTS

FACTORS

SLEEP

CAFFEINE

ALCOHOL

WATER

FOOD

WEATHER

OTHER FACTORS

NOTES

DATE

DURATION

INTENSITY

PAIN CHARACTERISTICS

TREATMENT

FACTORS

SLEEP

CAFFEINE

ALCOHOL

WATER

FOOD

WEATHER

NOTES

OTHER FACTORS

DATE

DURATION

INTENSITY

PAIN CHARACTERISTICS

TREATMENT

WHERE IT HURTS

FACTORS

SLEEP

CAFFEINE

ALCOHOL

WATER

FOOD

WEATHER

OTHER FACTORS

NOTES

www.ingramcontent.com/pod-product-compliance
Lightning Source LLC
Chambersburg PA
CBHW070747250726
48662CB00004B/1683